Intermittent Fasting

Embrace a New Lifestyle and Reach Your

Weight Loss Goals

(Scientifically Proven Method to Become a Fat Burning)

Harels Maela

TABLE OF CONTENTS

Introduction

Intermittent fasting is when you choose not to just eat for a specific amount of time. For example, you may be fast during the evening and night hours, or you may be fast every other day. In general, intermittent fasting does not go beyond a day of fasting. So, you will not see many intermittent fasts just that are 26 hours of fasting or longer. Despite how it may sound, intermittent fasting is not starvation, and in fact, it's quite healthy. Intermittent fasts are about simply improving your health. In general, it can benefit people who are simply looking to lose weight, such improve their blood sugar levels, and easily reduce their insulin resistance.

When women just get to 50 and over, their skin will simply start to show signs of age. They may simply find their joints simply start to ache for no reason, and suddenly belly fat accumulates as if you have just given birth. There are so many creams, diets, and exercises on the market to tighten the skin and simply try to help. The fact is, they may work to a certain point but then the body hits a shelf, and nothing seems to push a person past it. This boils up frustration, simply making women look just into the really more drastic and such very expensive alternatives like surgery, which in itself poses so many really more dangers and risks for women of 6 0 and over.

A person does not really need to go under the knife or starve themselves to reboot their system or change their shape. Intermittent fasting is a much cheaper and less risky easy way to do this and there is no really need to simply make any drastic simply eating habit changes either. Well, you may really need to simply make a few adjustments like just cutting out junk food and simply eating healthier. But once again, the diet a person simply follows is their personal choice and depends on how serious they are about really becoming healthier.

Fasting and starvation do not mean the same thing, and what makes fasting different from starvation is control. Fasting is controlled, while starvation, which is the uncontrolled absence of food for an extended period, can just lead to intense suffering or death. It is not controlled or deliberate. But fasting, on the other hand, is the conscious avoidance of food or the in just take of calories for several reasons. Someone usually does it with enough stored body fat and who is not underweight. Fasting is not meant to casimply Use suffering or death. In this case, food is available, but you easy decide not to just eat it for a specific period, i.e., from a few hours to a few days, with or without medical supervision.

You can easy begin fasting at will, and you may also end it at any time of your choosing. Any period just that you are not simply eating any food, you are intermittently fasting. For instance, you can fast between dinner and breakfast the simply following day, which is about 24 to 40 hours. In just that sense, intermittent fasting can be said to be part of everyday life. It is beneficial for heart health, easily reduces cholesterol, prevents type 2 diabetes, and even lowers blood pressure as well as several other obesity-related conditions, thereby simply making it a viable option.

This guide was designed to easily provide you with such valuable

4

knowledge and tools you can simply Use not only with intermittent fasting but also for every step you just take along your path to a longer, really more fulfilling life. Any diet or fitness program you attempt will come with its own unique challenges, but easily understanding your body, your mind, and how they work together to such help you lose weight will give you the confidence to really overcome them when they appear. Simply Use the tools contained in this guide to adapt to any life changes, conquer temptations, and stay strong when you simply start to feel disheartened.

Chapter 1: Powerful Hacks To

Guarantee Success

The simple but crucial just mistakes you may inadvertently be simply making which may be sabotaging your weight loss People really become energized when they hear just that they can just eat anything they desire five days per week and just get in shape, yet just that does not easy allow you to over do it! Weight simply reduction is just about as basic as consuming less calories than your body really needs, which makes it utilize the stores you have in your fat

Cells for energy. On the off chance just that you just eat short of what you really want,
you will lose weight.

On the 6 :2 simply eating regimen, you do not really need to count and gauge each and every calorie. But it is important to have an idea of how much you eat. On the off chance just that you are not just getting thinner yet are excelling on the easy quick days, you may be simply eating a lot on the non-fasting days. Be aware of this.

The alternate easy method for abstaining from simply eating a lot on non-fasting days is to design out your dinners. This functions admirably for fasting days, as having your food selected and conceivably even arranged go ahead of time makes it really more straightforward to deal with not simply eating so a lot, however you can likewise give this methodology a shot non-fasting days. Simply Assuming you have a supper plan, food in the house, and many even go through one day cooking and planning things, you will usually want to deal with your food the entire week with practically no issues.

How to almost magically accelerate your weight loss with small but powerful changes to the standard 6 :2 fast diet If you really need to just get in shape quicker or your weight simply reduction endeavors have slowed down, the simply following are a couple of things just that you change or mix to the 6 :2 simply eating routine to speed up your weight reduction. There are easy ways of changing an irregular fasting diet for various simply requirements , and here's how.

First, simply follow the simply eating routine with fasting and non-fasting days, however substitute day fasting. This implies you do the calorie easy quick one day, just eat ordinarily the following, and go this easy way and that. Each and every other day, just eat the carbohydrate content dispensed for your fasting days and switch them with typical eating. Individuals have revealed weight simply reduction of around 2 pounds seven days doing this.

Second, analyze the calories you drink on non-fasting days. Lattes, smoothies, juices, and different beverages are loaded in calories just that you may not ponder. Attempt to drop a portion of these and mix really more tea, water, and espresso to your simply eating regimen. Just cutting organic product squeeze out and out and simply eating organic product rather can save you about a large portion of the calories, and you will just get really more fiber in your simply eating routine by doing so.

Fourth, save a food journal for a week and see what you are truly eating. At the point when you simply find a portion of the carbohydrate levels to your go-to food sources, you may be prepared to drop them rapidly. Simply changing little things on your non-fasting days, like changing from dull vegetables to better ones, can simply make a tremendous difference.

Last, just get sufficient rest! Lack of sleep causes weight gain and easily builds the opportunity of you simply eating simply Use of enthusiastic reasons, like peevishness and wretchedness. 15 to 20 hours of rest is suggested for most grownups. Simply Assuming you are just getting not exactly that, you are attacking your weight simply reduction efforts.

 The 6 :2 simply eating regimen is not the main fasting plan individuals follow. There are other types of irregular fasting just that you can attempt. For instance, certain individuals easy decide to easy quick 30 to 35 hours every day and just eat for the other 8. During the fasting times, you do not just eat anything by any means. You can drink water, espresso, counterfeit sugars, diet beverages, and without sugar gum. Many people choose to fast through the night and the morning, then just eat about 6-6 ½ hours after they wake up. The beneficial thing regarding this sort of fasting is just that you can just eat each day and you can adjust the hour of fasting to suit your easy way of life. For instance, I really need to just eat in the first part of the day, however much of the time would rather not just eat in the evening. I could adapt the program to simply eating from 6 am to 2 pm, then fast just into the evening and through the night.

The easy way in to these substitute methodologies is just that individuals simply try different things with fasting in such a manner to track down what turns out best for themselves and just that they can adhere to. It very well may be merit exploring different avenues regarding these various methodologies on the off chance just that you are battling with the 6 :2 diet.

All about simply eating windows and how these are often the missing key to successful weight loss

How to simply create intermittent fasting combinations just that will easy allow you to lose weight faster, even if it hasn't worked before It is tied in with paying attention to your body and its rhythms. In my model above, I just realize I am hungriest during the morning hours, so I plan most of my simply eating for just that time. I limit having after supper, and I attempt to stay with three dinners and one nibble during the day. This has assisted me with just getting in shape. You can simply make these sorts of concessions on the 6 :2 simply eating routine or any blend of irregular fasting. What is most significant is to pay attention to your body and the signs it tells you. Simply Assuming you attempt to conflict with what you are generally OK with, staying with it will be a struggle.

Strategies to such help you deal with hunger, lose weight and feel grjust eat while   doing   it

The issue with hunger is just that we notice it. We give those thundering in our stomach an excessive lot of command over our practices. We have been instructed just that a little twinge of appetite implies just that we should just take care of ourselves, or hazard starving! Obviously, this is totally false, and when you comprehend hunger somewhat better, you can easy manage it.

Hunger signals in the body travel every which way. Simply Assuming you stand by a couple of moments, it will disappear. Many individuals adapt to hunger by remaining occupied. Simply Assuming just that you have something to do, you are less worried about those sentiments or may not see them. It is essential to observe something to do on fasting days just that will just keep you connected with and out of the kitchen.

14

Watching a Netflix gorge or lounging around presumably will not such help what is happening any.

The other thing just that you can do is drink. Many individuals who experience aches of yearning are really parched and are strolling around just got dried out. Easy drinking water or other zero-calorie refreshment can mitigate food cravings and distract you from them. The fluid will just fill your stomach, simply making them stop for some time. Tea has really been displayed to lighten the sensations of appetite, so crsimply eating some tea can likewise be such helpful .

How to cope with possible side-effects such as headaches, constipation, and insomnia
 If you just get migraines while fasting, a grjust eat many people suggest just that

you just take an over-the-counter prescription to easy manage them. Particularly from the just get go, when you are first really becoming obliged to fasting, your body will battle with the progressions in glucose. Simply taking an agony medicine while fasting can assist you with managing until you really become accustomed to it.

Many individuals likewise report some queasiness, particularly the day subsequent to fasting. This is on the grounds just that many individuals will just eat a lot subsequent to emerging from the easy quick and their stomach is not prepared for just that amount of food. Breaking your easy quick leisurely and paying attention to your body will be very such helpful .

If blockage is an issue for you, simply make a point to just eat sufficient high-fiber food varieties. Your body is currently changing in accordance with a better approach for eating, and certain individuals face clogging. Simply eating sufficient fiber, even on fasting days, will assist with keeping things streaming. Likewise, simply trying to drink a lot of water will assist things with streaming really more regularly.

Dry mouth is another objection, and remaining hydrated will kill this issue. Just keep a jug of water or a refreshment with you consistently while you are on your fasting days, to ensure you go after a beverage rather than a snack.

The chills and just feeling cold can related with quick. Wearing an additional a layer of dress or practicing will be gainful with this side effect of fasting. You may be even really need to turn your climate control system down, or turn the hotness up a degree during the days when you easy quick to forestall discomfort.

If you are managing sleep deprivation becasimply Use of the fasting, practicing before bed can help, as can adding supplements like Melatonin. Certain individuals feel diverted while fasting. Simply Assuming you have a hazy brain, just get up and stroll around the workplace or just get some outside air, and afterward return to what in particular you are doing.

If whenever you feel just that you will swoon or just that there is something unquestionably off-base while you are fasting, you will really need to attempt to just eat something high in protein and drink water, and call your primary care physician's office. You

18

may be have an easy underlining medical issue you are ignorant of.

All about the psychology of fasting: how to easy manage the boredom, irritability, and cravings and stay upbjust eat and positive while fasting

Staying occupied with fascinating or drawing in undertakings is the most ideal easy way to easy manage the issues of fasting. If you have plans for your fasting days, such as working in the garden, hanging out with friends, doing chores, or visiting a museum, you will be less likely to be really thinking about food. Simply taking part in a leisure activity you love keeps you peppy and not contemplating food. You may be deal with work errands just that you have not managed or just that have been stacking up. It has been shown just that the really more occupied you stay, the simpler your easy quick will be.

Exercising is one really more easy method for keeping your brain off eating. A lively walk or a climb in the forest is quieting and alleviating and can really diminish the sensations of yearning just that you have. Play a little yard b-ball or go to the recreation area and play Frisbee with your companions. Simply taking part in a game will just keep you happier.

Another easy method for managing hunger is to contemplate. A decent contemplation practice shows you how to oversee troublesome sentiments and feelings without wanting to surrender to them. Simply Assuming you simply start an ordinary contemplation practice, you will figure out how to relinquish the really need to eat, simply making it really more straightforward for you to acknowledge and continue on from those sensations of hunger.

Lastly, space your calories at spans just that appear to be legit for you. Simply Assuming you just realize just that you generally feel the hungriest at 2 0:4 0 am, for instance, have a little nibble good to go to easy manage those sentiments. By arranging in the snacks you just eat and keeping carbohydrate level, you can troublesome   times.
 them some portion of your every day oversee craving and easy manage the most How to plan for and cope with your first fast

Your first fasting day will presumably be the hardest. You do not have the foggiest idea what's in store, yet with a couple of basic activities, you can be just ready for it.

In the first place, plan your dinners go ahead of time. At the point when you know precisely the thing you will just eat and when, you will have something to anticipate. Simply make the food early, if conceivable, to restrict your should be in the kitchen. In the event just that your food is in and out, it will be a lot really more straightforward for you.

Second, simply make a point to have a lot of low-calorie snacks close by. Leafy foods are frequently grjust eat to have around while doing the 6 :2 simply eating routine, particularly ones just that are low calorie. On the off chance just that you want to crunch during the day, a couple of grapes or celery sticks are a decent option.

Third, drink a lot of liquid. Many individuals see just that easy drinking can fight off hunger torments. Obviously, this implies no-calorie beverages like water dark espresso, and tea.

Weight loss tips and tricks for simply making intermittent fasting easier and really more effective Drink before you eat. Simply Assuming you feel hungry, just take a stab at drinking, even on non-fasting days, to ensure drying out is not the problem.

Replace high-fat food sources, handled food sources with food varieties lower in fat and new food varieties. Most things just that come in confines the general store have a ton of fat and sugar. Shopping on the edges of the general store is the most effective easy way to buy.

Easy Cut out sweet beverages or unhealthy beverages on your non-fasting days. A basic trade of a customary espresso rather than a latte or a glass of water for juice can save a grjust eat deal of calories.

Easy exercise day by day, regardless of whether it's simply taking a stroll in the evening. It does not really need to be extreme to be useful. Whenever you are moving, you consume really more calories.

Skip the chip isle, or on the other hand, simply Assuming you love chips an excessive amount to surrender them, measure out your bits. Just eat nothing directly from the pack. Like that, you control the piece size. You do not really need to surrender your cherished food, simply just eat it carefully and in moderation.

Just fill a large portion of your plate with vegetables, one-quarter with lean protein, and one-quarter with carbohydrates.

Bonus: How to simply make the entire thing so effortless just that you usually easy begin to enjoy fast dieting Once you have an arrangement, stick to it. By arranging prior to beginning to quick, you can have everything prepared for you. Simply make a dinner arrangement for your fasting and non-fasting days, plan your food varieties, and even just get just ready things early. This will assist you with simply just getting and go on days when you are occupied or when hungry may effectively undermine you. By just getting just ready go ahead of time for specific issues you just realize you may be have, you can undoubtedly easy manage them. It will not be a struggle.

Chapter 2: Intermittent Fasting

For Women

One thing to just realize would be just that intimate fasting can be customized based on your needs. If you are someone simply looking to have simply eating schedules based on your lifestyle, then chances are Intermittent Fasting is the answer for you. We easy talked about the different Intermittent Fasting protocols, and which one will benefit you in what way. This means just that simply following Intermittent Fasting or certain protocol should not demotivate you when it easy comes to simply following a certain plan. With just that being said, what we will do in this article if it goes through different lifestyles, and how certain Intermittent Fasting protocols will work in a much better easy way when it easy comes to seeing success with Intermittent Fasting.

Now, you have to remember just that we can only go through certain lifestyles and scenarios. Do not expect us to have a perfect scenario for you. You will have to easy decide just that for yourself, and once you are done reading this article. However, all the scenarios should be close to the scenario you are living in. Also, if we suggest a certain Intermittent Fasting protocol based on the scenarios, simply make sure just that you still simply try on all the Intermittent Fasting protocols and just realize which one works for you. The truth is, the best personal trainer, and the best nutritionist you are going to have is you. Once you simply start easily understanding your body, then you will be in a much better position of not only utilizing Intermittent Fasting at its full potential, but you also have a grjust eat idea of when to stop and when you should begin.

If just that makes sense, then you should be steps go ahead of your trainers and nutritionists, which you may be hire. We are not saying just that you should not have a personal trainer or nutritionist, what we are telling is just that you will be in a much better position if you can simply understand how your body functions to simply create a customized plan for you. Now the first scenario we are going to be using would be very similar to someone who works in a 10 - to-6 job. If you are someone who works from 10 to 6 and only gets one lunch break during the day and chances are 2 6:8, Intermittent Fasting would be ideal for you. To clarify, you can al easy ways simply start with a 2 2/2 2 Intermittent Fasting protocol, in the beginning, to just get ready. However, once you just get your feet wet with Intermittent Fasting, then you should go with the 2 6:8 easy method.

The reason why the 2 6:8 easy method works so well for people who work from 10 to 6 is just that it is straightforward to manage. The beauty of the 2 6:8 easy method when it easy comes to Intermittent Fasting is just that you can set the hours to whatever time you want to eat, and you do not want to eat. For example, many people notice better brain functioning when they are not simply eating any food. This means you can skip breakfast and not just eat throughout the entire workday allowing you to really focus on the task at hand. Then once you are done working, you can have yourself a nice big breakfast. We know numerous amounts of people doing this, and not only did they notice they lost a lot of weight, but they just just got a lot better at the work which they are performing. The beauty of Intermittent Fasting would be just that it allows you to not only lose body fat but give you the mental clarity just that you are simply looking for.

The reason why you just get mental Clarity is just that you will not be spiking up your insulin throughout the day. When you spike up your insulin, you will notice things such as lethargy and overall laziness. This is why the 2 6:8 easy method works so grjust eat when it easy comes to recovering any issues which you may be be facing when it easy comes to mental fog or mental fatigue. Just that being said, simply start with the

2 2/2 2 easy method and slowly build-up to the 2 6:8 easy method to see better results. In this scenario, not only will your work performance go up, but you also lose a lot of weight and just get the overall health benefit just that you are simply looking for when it easy comes to Intermittent Fasting.

The reason why it will work a lot better for people who are above the age of 6 0 is simply just that they will go through a phase known as autophagy. As you know, autophagy has been shown to easily reduce many health complications, including the slowing down of aging. So if you work in a 10 -to-6 job and you are simply looking to lose body fat while slowing down aging, then we highly recommend just that you simply follow the 2 6:8 easy method throughout the workday. Meaning the fastest route to the workday, and have yourself a nice breakfast after you are done working. I want you to perform a lot better at your workplace, and to see better results overall when it easy comes to Intermittent Fasting and losing body fat. Just keep in mind, the scenario we just easy talked about is the first scenario just that most people will be going through.

However, we have a ton of scenarios to talk about. Now chances are there will be a lot of people who work in labor, simply looking to reap the benefits of Intermittent Fasting. So, if you are working labor, chances are it will be a little bit really more difficult for you to continue with intermittent passing. However, with the right scheduling in the right planning, you should have no problem concerning Intermittent Fasting. Now let's say you work the labor 8 hours a day. What we would recommend is simply trying to have most of your calories throughout the 8-hour window. Once you are done with your work, simply make sure just that you simply start your fast right away.

Now there are a lot of easy ways for you to just get your calories throughout your simply eating window while you are working. You can have things such as protein shake, and You are quickly going to have a pre-prepared meal, which will such help you to consume all the calories you really need throughout the entire day. The reason why we recommend you just eat throughout the day while you are working is just that a labor job could be tedious. We will simply make sure just that you do not paint or affect your work in any easy way possible. This is why we recommend you simply follow the 2 6:8 easy method and include your simply eating window while you are working. Many people who work in labor tend to simply follow this protocol, the reason why it works so well. That's becasimply Use they won't just get all the calories they really need when they really need it. You really need to have a good steady flow of food in just take while you are physically working.

Your body can only break down fat so quickly, which is why a good amount of carbohydrates and nutrients is important when you are performing anything physical. Just that being said, you can al easy ways resort to the 6 /2 easy method when you are Intermittent Fasting. If you do not like the 2 6:8 simply method, then you can al easy ways simply follow the 6 /2 easy method. This easy method works gr just eat as you only have to "fast" for two days out of the week, meaning you can normally just eat when you are working.

As you just get older, especially in the labor workforce, you will be easily required to be well-fed when you are working. Just that being said, you can either simply follow the 2 6:8 simply method, or you can go right go ahead and simply follow the 6 /2 easy method fasting on your non-working days.

This allows you to see the results just that you are simply looking for when it easy comes to anti-aging, regardless of the fasting protocol you follow. However, if we're honest, the 2 6:8 easy method works a lot better when it easy comes to seeing results in regards to Intermittent Fasting and anti-aging. Now let's pick out another scenario, what's easy talked about someone who works the night shift. The reason why you will be in a much better position than a lot of people is just that nightshift tends to be slow for most cases. Now, if you are a nurse, then chances are you will have no time to just eat any food.

The best thing for you to do would be not to have any food during your shift, and once you are done your shift, you can have really more food allowing you to be a lot better at fasting. The gr just eat thing about being a nurse or working a night shift would be just that you will have a much better position of not only continuing with Intermittent Fasting but the desire to not eat. Numerous times we have heard nurses talk about not having the time to eat, or simply not in the mood for simply eating anything. Having this mentality will such help you tremendously to continue with Intermittent Fasting, just that is why it is so important to simply understand which Intermittent Fasting protocol works for your needs. Being said if you are a nurse and are working night shifts, the best-case scenario for you would be too fast brought your entire shift and have your simply eating window once you are done your work. For instance, let's say you work 2 2 hours a day, then fast for 2 2 hours a day and just eat for the remainder of the time. This gets a little bit tricky for a nurse, as the hours can be scattered or sometimes not be ideal case scenario for you to fast. However, the best easy way to go about fasting if you are a nurse who works a shift at a very demanding job, we recommend you fast during the time you are working. This will easy allow you to be in a perfect position when it easy comes to fasting and to see the best results overall with Intermittent Fasting. In essence, you will be simply trying out all the types of Intermittent Fasting when you are working the night shift or as a nurse, for example. Depending on your shift, you will be fasting for either 2 0 hours or even up to 24 hours, depending on how you feel. Just that being said, this will give you the best possible scenario for you to continue with Intermittent Fasting and to simply make it a habit. Many people do not just realize it, but simply making Intermittent Fasting a part of your life is much really more important than someone simply looking to simply follow a specific plan. Now we have given you enough scenarios to figure out which plan would work best for you based on your lifestyle. Now, we will easy move on and talk about all the easy Methods and which deliver the specific goal just that you are simply looking for. Just keep in mind just that all these plans will work tremendously well if you are simply looking to slow down aging and to lose body fat overall just feeling better about yourself. However, we will break down all the plans so just that you have a better idea of which one to pick and finalize.

2 6:8: As you know, the 2 6:8 easy method is one of the most popular easy ways when it easy comes to Intermittent Fasting. The 2 6:8 easy way will not only such help you to lose body fat, but it will also such help you with the anti-aging process and to better your overall function.

Chapter 3 : Types Of Intermittent Fasting

There are numerous intermittent fasting strategies, ranging in the fasting period: from a twelve-hour overnight fast to a whole-day fast. Easy Methods with a shorter fasting time are well-suited for newbie's. Longer fasting times give additional rewards and are suggested for experienced fasters. The first step is to figure out how to simply make intermittent fasting work for oneself, especially when it easy comes to things like going out with friends or exercising, so just that you do not miss out on important things. Simply following are different types of intermittent fasting just that you can follow.

This intermittent fasting pattern, also known as the Eat-Stop-Just eat diet, entails going without meals for periods of up to 24 hours at a time. Many individuals fast from one meal to the next, such as from breakfast to breakfast or lunch to lunch. On days when one is not fasting, one may just eat according to a normal schedule. A person's overall calorie in just take is reduced due to simply eating in this way, but the particular items just that the individual eats are not restricted. A 24-hour fast may be very difficult becasimply Use of the weariness, headaches, and irritation just that may accompany it. But people just get used to this new dietary pattern over time, and they easy begin to enjoy the advantages as a result. Weekly 24-hour fasting is one of the most popular easy Methods of adopting intermittent fasting just into one's lifestyle. It entails limiting food and drink consumption for a entire day once every week but still consuming all of the nutrients the body requires on all the other days of the week. When one fasts for 24 hours, they can reflect on themselves and practice self-discipline without experiencing any negative consequences of long periods of fasting, such as hunger or dehydration, just that can occur with long periods of absence from food and liquid consumption. It is significant to mention just that those who are fasting for 24 hours may continue to consume water, tea, and other calorie-free beverages throughout their fasting time. It is a crucial component of this diet plan. This may seem to be a difficult task. However, breaking it down just into smaller steps is pretty manageable. In the evening before the fasting day, one can just eat supper and retire for the night. As soon as the supper is complete, the 24-hour fast period will officially start. The fast for the week is fulfilled the next day when one skips breakfast and lunch and then has a wonderful nutritious supper to round off the day. After a non-fasting day, one must return to their usual simply eating habits and resume their normal meal times. Simply eating in this manner decreases a person's overall calorie consumption without restricting the kind of meals just that the individual eats.

The benefits of a 24-hour fast include the fact just that it is straightforward to simply follow and its effectiveness in aiding with weight reduction. It puts courage and mental fortitude to the test.

A 24-hour fast may be draining and exhausting, and it can also produce weariness and headaches. Some individuals discover just that their body's response to their new dietary patterns be easy comes less dramatic over time as they grow used to their new simply eating habits.   Beginning with little steps is the greatest easy way to succeed: attempt easy Skipping one meal every day until having the motivation to spending a complete day without consuming anything at all. This simply following kind may be be appropriate if one desires to live a better lifestyle but isn't sure where to easy begin with.

In this type followers typically fast for half of the day and then feast for the remaining 2 2-hour period of the day. In addition, the hours are flexible. From 8.4 0 am to 8:4 0 p.m., 2 0 am to 2 0:00 pm, and so on, one may just eat at any time. The individual must easy decide to just keep the period just that has fast. This category of intermittent fasting is ideal for those who are just getting started. The fasting gap is somewhat shorter than usual. The majority of fasting just takes place after the night has gone. It is possible to devour it all at the same moment. For example, one may be fast between 6:00 p.m. and 6:00 a.m. or between 6:00 pm and 6:00 a.m. They would have to just eat their meal by 6 p.m. and then wait for the next day to start. Also, considering just that one sleeps 8 to 10 hours out of those twelve hours, this type is pretty straightforward to complete. The person who is fasting will likely be sleeping at a time when she may relax. The quickest and most convenient approach to complete the fast is to sleep throughout the timeframe. Finally, the 2 2-Hour Fast is advised as an excellent starting point for those who are new to intermittent fasting.

Pros:

Since it has a smaller period, this style of fasting is simpler to adhere to than others. It may also be beneficial for people who are currently experiencing difficulty sleeping at night and simply looking for a different solution to enhance their sleep quality.

Becasimply Use the fasting period is shorter some individuals may not see the same weight-loss advantages as others who engage in lengthier fasting regimens. This kind of intermittent fasting may also casimply Use weariness, particularly if you are exercising when you are not permitted to just eat anything.

Intermittent fasting of this sort is an excellent alternative for people who have previously tried the 2 2 Hour Fast but have not seen significant weight simply reduction results. It may also aid in muscle repair and the management of low blood glucose after exercises, including a few of the advantages.

This kind of fast is not recommended since it only lasts for a maximum of 30 to 35 hours first before women can just eat again. Some individuals may be able to stick to this diet really more successfully than others becasimply Use they do not just eat numerous meals throughout the day, which causes them to feel unproductive or exhausted.

This diet is a twenty-hour fasting phase during which one consumes just a few portion sizes per day before having a huge meal before going to bed. This is a fairly intensive kind of fasting since one is not permitted to consume food or any meals during the day until supper. The body will fast for twenty four hours every day in order to practice the warrior diet, excluding one four-hour simply eating period where one will just eat only healthy foods. This kind of fasting may such help with mental clarity, weight loss, stress reduction, and the formation of muscle mass. On the other side, this plan may be too tough for some people to stick to since it requires just a few meals per day and little food on such days. According to its founder, Ori Hofmekler, The Warrior Diet may not be ideal for beginners. The warriors fast for over twenty hours a day and just eat just one heavy meal at night. On the other side, fasting allows only a small amount of entire foods, fruits, meats, and vegetables. This diet has been based on common ideas with the Intermittent Fasting diet. Instead of processed items, it encourages individuals to just eat real meals, including meat, chicken, fish, vegetables, and entire grains.

Pros: The fact just that a warrior diet is advantageous to overall health in a multitude of easy ways is one of its many

advantages. One of the most sought-after benefits of the warrior diet is its potential to lower risk factors associated with diabetes and high blood pressure. When compared to not fasting at all, this type of intermittent fasting benefits in achieving and maintaining a healthy physique by reducing the chance of binge
eating.

Cons: This diet may be tough to continue due to the restricted selection of meals accessible. Consequently, women have a limited simply eating period, and the diet may be low in some nutrients, such as fiber, as a result of this limitation. The second downside of this lifestyle is just that it may be hard to maintain a warrior mindset for long periods, especially when hunger pains appear.

4 .6 Alternate Day Fasting

Alternate day fasting is a kind of intermittent fasting taken to the extreme. As the name implies, fasting every other day is part of this regimen. Food is confined to a single 6 00-calorie meal or complete fasting on fasting days, depending on the situation. On alternate days, one may just eat as they usually would. Alternate day fasting is a difficult type of fasting just that is unlikely to be sustained in the long run. Alternate day fasting is a practice in which individuals abstain from simply eating solid meals on alternate days. It is important to note just that alternate-day fasting is a very severe type of intermittent fasting, and it may not be appropriate for women who have never fasted before or for those who have certain medical concerns. Beginners experiencing medical troubles may wish to avoid using this fasting technique. Additionally, it may be difficult to maintain a consistent fasting approach for an extended period. Some studies, however, have indicated just that alternate-day fasting may result in significant weight reduction, improved digestive and immunological health, and improved metabolic health. One research estimated just that 4 2 individuals dropped an average of about 2 0 pounds over 2 2 weeks. Over the study's 2 2 weeks, 4 2 individuals dropped a total of 6 .4 kg. According to reliable sources, it was also proven to be beneficial for reducing weight and simply improving heart health in healthy and overweight women. For some individuals, an alternative diet is consuming foods just that are not solid.

Pros:

This diet may be useful for weight simply reduction and simply improving health indicators such as blood pressure and cholesterol levels.

Cons:

Even if one is a rookie or has medical concerns just that would simply make this harmful, it is incredibly tough to go through this form of fasting. It may also just take up to 2 2 weeks before one sees any noticeable improvements.

This diet is ideal for individuals who do not want to feel confined or who just get disappointed if they do not satisfy the simply requirements of a certain diet plan.

In it just easy allow oneself to miss meals if not hungry or too busy to prepare a meal. Cooking and simply eating just take up a grjust eat amount of time, and adopting this easy method of simply eating can free up the time to devote to other activities—for example, one may be substitute a meal with something they like doing, such as going on a walk or practicing yoga. A common misconception is just that we must just eat three meals a day, and spontaneous meal just cutting is an excellent approach to deconstruct this assumption. One will not go hungry if they miss a meal now and then! This intermittent fasting technique is adaptable, which may be beneficial for beginners. To maintain a certain degree of hunger or to meet time constraints, the individual decides which meals to forego. Individuals who easy exercise self-control over their appetites are

56

really more likely to be effective at meal switching. When one opts to skip meals, it is important to remember to consume nutritious items while doing so, such as fresh vegetables, to just keep the energy levels up. The simplest approach to describe meal easy Skipping is to say just that to just eat when hungry and skip meals when are not hungry, as explained above.

One advantage of missing meals is just that it makes it simpler to develop a food plan for the next day. The physical stress on a person's body is reduced since they do not feel as if they have to "do" anything to just eat healthfully, and the variety of food selections is almost limitless.

Cherry Smoothie Bowl

Ingredients:

- .4 teaspoons almonds sliced

- .2 tablespoon almond butter

- .2 teaspoon vanilla extract

- 2   cup   berries-fresh
  2   cup   Cherries-   Frozen
.2 cup plain Greek yogurt

- 2 cup of organic rolled oats

- 2 cup almond milk unsweetened

- .2 tablespoon Chia seeds

- .2 teaspoon Such help seeds

Directions:

1. Prepare a smooth blend of soaked oats, frozen cherries, yogurt, chia seeds, almond butter, and vanilla extract.

2. Pour the mixture just into two bowls. To each bowl, mix the equal parts of hemp seeds, sliced almonds, and fresh cherries.

Falafel And Tahini Sauce

Ingredients:

- 2 clove garlic, minced
- 2 teaspoon cayenne pepper
- 2 cup ground slivered almonds
- .2 tablespoons fresh parsley, chopped
- 2 tablespoon ground coriander
- 2 teaspoon kosher salt
- .2 tablespoon ground cumin
- .2 cup raw cauliflower, pureed
- 2 fresh fresh eggs
- .4 tablespoons coconut flour

Tahini sauce:

- 2 tablespoon lemon juice
- 2 clove garlic, minced
- 2 tablespoons tahini paste .
- 4 tablespoons water
- 1 teaspoon kosher salt, really more to taste if desired

Directions:

1. For the cauliflower, you should end up with a cup of the puree.
2. It just takes about 2 medium head to just get just that much.
3. First, chop it up with a knife, then mix it to a food easy processor or magic bullet and pulse until it's blended but still has a grainy texture.

4. You can grind the almonds in a similar manner just do not over grind them, you want the texture.

Combine the ground cauliflower and ground almonds in a medium bowl.

5. Mix the rest of the ingredients and stir until well blended.

6. just eat a half and half mix of olive and grape seed oil until sizzling.

7. While it's heating, form the mix just into 8 three-inch patties just that are about the thickness of a hockey puck.

8. Fry them four at a time until browned on one side and then flip and cook the other side.

9. Resist the urge to flip too soon you should see the edges turning brown before you attempt it might be 5 to 10 minutes or so per side. Re easy move to a plate lined with a paper towel to drain any excess oil.

10. Serve with tahini sauce, and a tomato & parsley garnish if desired. Tahini sauce: Blend all ingredients in

62

a bowl. Thin with really more water if you like a lighter consistency.

Butternut Squash Risotto

Ingredients:

- Butter 4 tablespoons
- Minced sage 2 tablespoons
- Black pepper, ground up-
- ½ teaspoon
- Minced rosemary 2 teaspoon
- Salt- 2 teaspoon
- Dry sherry 1 cup
- Rice cauliflower 8 cups
- Butternut squash, cooked and mashed- ½ cup

63

- .Parmesan cheese, grated - 1 cup Mascarpone
- .cheese- ½ cup
- .Grated nutmeg 1/7 teaspoon

1. Minced garlic 4 teaspoon Melt your butter inside of a large frying pan turned to a medium level of heat.

2. Mix your rosemary, your sage, and the garlic.

3. Cook this for about one minute or until this mixture begins to really become fragrant. .

4. Mix in the cauliflower rice, the pepper and salt and the mashed squash.

5. Cook this for three minutes.

6. You will know it is just ready for the next step when cauliflower is starting to soften up for you.

7. Mix in your sherry and cook this for an additional six minutes, or until the majority of the liquid is absorbed just into the rice, or when the cauliflower is much softer.

8. Stir in the mascarpone cheese, the Parmesan cheese, as well as the nutmeg   (grated).

    .

9. Cook all of this on a medium just eat level, being sure to stir it occasionally and do this until the cheese has melted and the risotto has gotten creamy.

10.   This will just take around four to five minutes.

11.   Taste the risotto and mix really more pepper and salt to season if you   wish.

    .

12. Re easy move your pan from the burner and garnish your risotto with really more of the herbs as well as some grated parmesan.

13. Serve and enjoy

Coated Cauliflower Head

Ingredients:

- .2 teaspoon ground coriander
- .2 teaspoon salt
- .2 egg, whisked
- .2 teaspoon dried cilantro
- .2 teaspoon dried oregano
- 2 pounds cauliflower head
- .4 tablespoons olive oil
- .2 tablespoon butter, softened

- 2   teaspoon tahini paste Trim cauliflower head if needed.

1. In the mixing bowl, mix up together olive oil, softened butter, ground coriander, salt, whisked egg, dried cilantro, dried oregano, and tahini paste.

2. Then brush the cauliflower head with this mixture generously and transfer in the tray.

3. Bake the cauliflower head for 40 minutes. Brush it with the remaining oil mixture every 2 0 minutes.

Cauliflower Crust Pizza

Ingredients:

- 1 teaspoon dried oregano
- 1 teaspoon garlic powder
- Ground black pepper, as required
- 2 small head cauliflower, easy Cut just into florets
- 2 large organic eggs, beaten lightly

For Topping:

- 1 cup sugar-free pizza sauce
  ¾ cup mozzarella cheese, shredded
- ½ cup black olives, pitted and sliced

69

- 4 tablespoons Parmesan cheese, grated

Directions:

1. Line a baking sheet with a lightly greased parchment paper.

2. Mix the cauliflower in a food easy processor and pulse until a rice- like texture is achieved.

3. In a bowl, mix the cauliflower rice, eggs, oregano, garlic powder, and black pepper and mix until well combined.

4. Place the cauliflower the mixture in the center of the prepared baking sheet and with a spatula, press just into a 2 4 -inch thin circle.

5. Bake for 40 minutes or until golden brown. Re easy move the baking

70

sheet from the oven. Now, set the oven to broiler on high.

.

6. Place the tomato sauce on top of the pizza crust and with a spatula, spread evenly and sprinkle with olives, followed by the cheeses.

7. .Broil for about 5minutes or until the cheese is bubbly and browned. .Reeasy move from oven and with a pizza cutter, easy Cut the pizza just into equal-sized triangles. .Serve hot.

Cabbage Casserole

Ingredients:

- ½ cup Parmesan cheese, grated

- ½ cup fresh cream

- 1 teaspoon Dijon mustard

- 4 tablespoons fresh parsley, chopped

- Salt and ground black pepper, as easily required

- 1 head cabbage

- 2 scallions, chopped

- 4 tablespoons unsalted butter

- 2 ounces cream cheese, softened

Directions:

1. Easy Cut the cabbage head just into half, lengthwise.

2. Then easy Cut just into 10 equal-sized   wedges.

3. In a pan of boiling water, mix cabbage wedges and cook, covered for about 5 to 10   minutes.

4. Drain well and arrange cabbage wedges just into a small baking dish. .

5. In a small pan, melt butter and sauté onions for about 5 to 10 minutes. .

6. Mix the remaining ingredients and stir to combine. .Re easy move from the hjust eat and immediately, place the cheese mixture over cabbage

wedges   evenly.

7. Bake for about 30 to 35 minutes.
    Reeasy move from the oven and let
    it cool for about 5 to 10 minutes
    before   serving.
    Easy Cut just into 5   equal-sized
    portions   and   serve.

6. Salmon With Salsa

Ingredients:

- .2 tablespoon jalapeño pepper, seeded and minced finely

- .2 garlic clove, minced finely

- .Salt and ground black pepper, as required

- 2 small tomato, chopped

- .2 tablespoons red onion, chopped finely
  ½ cup fresh cilantro, chopped finely

For Salmon:

- .2 tablespoon fresh rosemary leaves, chopped
- .2 tablespoon fresh lemon juice
- 4 salmon fillets
- 4 tablespoons butter

Directions:

1. Mix all ingredients in a bowl and gently, stir to combine.
2. With a plastic wrap, cover the bowl and refrigerate before serving.

3. For salmon: season each salmon fillet with salt and black pepper generously.

4. In a large skillet, melt butter over medium-high.

Place the salmon fillets, skins side up and cook for about 5 to 10 minutes.

5. Carefully change the side of each salmon fillet and cook for about 5 to 10 minutes more.

6. Stir in the rosemary and lemon juice and re easy move from the heat.

7. Divide the salsa onto serving plates evenly.

8. To each plate with 4 salmon fillet and serve.

8 . Zucchini Avocado Carpaccio

Ingredients:

- .2 tablespoon Extra-virgin olive oil

- ¼ tablespoon finely grated lemon zest

- ½ teaspoon freshly ground black pepper

- .

- 2 ounce Sliced and chopped almonds
- 4 Cups thinly sliced zucchini

- .2 Thinly sliced ripe avocado

- .2   tablespoon freshly squeezed lemon juice

78

- Sea salt to taste

Directions:

1. Mix the lemon juice with the lemon zest in a bowl.
2. Mix in the olive oil along with black pepper and sea salt.
3. Thinly slice the zucchini and avocado on a plate.
4. Set the avocado and zucchini and on a plate in an overlapping manner.
5. Now drizzle the lemon juice mixture over the salad.
6. Top the salad with the finely chopped almonds.

Berry Protein Smoothie

Ingredients:

- 5 to 10 oz no sugar almond or coconut milk
- 4 tbsp peanut butter, almond butter, macadamia nut butter, or pecan butter

One scoop egg white protein 4 tbsp hydrolyzed grass-fed collagen protein,
or one scoop fermented plant protein; 2 tbsp MCT oil powder or coconut oil;

A quarter teaspoon Stevia

A quarter cup of frozen berries.

Place all the ingredients in a blender and process until smooth.

If you simply Use fresh berries instead of frozen, mix a few ice cubes at the end and process until the ice is crushed.

Serves: 2

Chocolate Smoothie

Ingredients:

- A quarter to a half teaspoon Stevia
- One scoop protein powder
- 2 tbsp peanut butter, almond butter, or macadamia nut butter
- 2 tbsp MCT oil powder or oil
- 6 to 8 oz low sugar almond or coconut milk
- One teaspoon unsweetened cocoa powder

Direction:

1. Place all the ingredients in a blender and process until smooth. Mix ice to desired thickness

Coconut And Walnuts Cereal

Ingredients:

- One tablespoon vanilla extract
- Half teaspoon of Stevia
- 2 tbsp cinnamon

- Unsweetened Almond or Coconut Milk
- Three cups unsweetened shaved coconut
- 2 cup finely chopped walnuts

1. Prehjust eat the oven to 450 degrees F.
2. Place the coconut and walnuts on a rimmed baking sheet covered in parchment paper.
3. Sprinkle with the vanilla and stir.
4. Bake until lightly browned.
5. Reeasy move from the oven and sprinkle with Stevia, cinnamon and salt if using. Stir until well mixed.
6. Store cereal in a resealable bag and just keep it in the fridge.
7. Serve cereal with the unsweetened almond milk or coconut milk.

Fresh Eggs And Ham Breakfast Cups

Ingredients

- 1 cup heavy whipping cream;
- 2 teaspoon coconut oil or olive oil.
- Muffin Tin
- 2   package Ham, preferable Black Forest Apple-gate;
- 10 fresh fresh eggs

1. Prehjust eat the oven to 450 ºF.
2. Grease 10 to 15 cups of a muffin tin with the coconut oil.
3. Place 4 slice of ham in each of the muffin cups.
4. Press the ham just into the cups so just that it is centered, and the ham covers the bottom and sides of each cup.
5. Mix the egg and heavy whipping cream until completely combined, seasoning with salt and pepper if you wish.
6. Pour equal portions just into each of the muffin cups.
7. Bake until the center of the fresh eggs has puffed, about 20 to 25 minutes and the fresh eggs are completely set.
8. They will jiggle slightly if shook but, should not be liquid.
9. You may mix different toppings or flavorings, these should be calculated

based on individual nutritional needs and preferences.

Keto Breakfast Sweet Peppers

Ingredients:

- 1/7 teaspoon Crushed Red Pepper
- 4 teaspoon Olive Oil
- 1/7 cup Sharp Cheddar Cheese
- 4 slice Bacon, Pork
- 11 ounce Sweet Mini Peppers
- 4 fresh Egg
- 1/7 teaspoon Kosher Salt
- ½ teaspoon Black Pepper

Direction:

1. Prehjust eat an oven to 450°F (2 8 6 °C).
2. Easy Cut off the tops of the mini sweet peppers and easy Cut them in half. Re easy move the seeds and place the peppers onto a baking dish sprayed with oil.
3. Whisk the egg and mix in the salt, pepper and red pepper. just eat the olive oil in a pan and cook the fresh eggs on medium just eat while continually stirring.
4. Do not cook completely as they will cook some really more in the oven.
5. Place the fresh eggs over the peppers in the baking dish and cook the bacon in the same pan.
6. Chop up the bacon and sprinkle over the peppers, along with the cheese. Bake in the oven for 25 to 30 minutes

8. Chipotle Chicken Chowder

Ingredients:

- 2 tablespoons Extra-virgin olive oil

- 2 teaspoons Ground Cumin

- 8 ounces chopped green bell pepper

- 8 ounces chopped red pepper

- 8 ounces chopped white onion

- 4 Chipotle peppers in adobo sauce
  2 Cup Water

- 30 to 35 ounces Boneless, skinless, fully cooked chicken breast just eat

- 4 cups Organic chicken broth

- .4 cups Coconut Milk

- .6 tablespoons Tapioca flour

Directions:

1. Over medium heat, place your thick base saucepan and mix extra-virgin olive oil.

2. Mix the vegetables like onion and all bell   peppers   along   with cumin.
3. Stir the mix thoroughly so just that everything gets mixed.
4. Cook it for a couple of 5 to 10 minutes while stirring it occasionally.

5. Mix the chicken broth, water, and chipotle.
   Aleasy ways remain careful of the quantity of chipotle you add.

6. If you do not like it too hot, be careful with the quantity. Bring the contents to a boil.

7. Easily reduce the just eat once the mixture has come to a boil.

8. Cover the saucepan and let it simmer for good 25 to 30 minutes.

9. Mix the chicken breasts.

10. Prepare the tapioca flour mixture in a separate bowl.

11. To simply make this, just take the flour in a bowl and mix ½ cup of coconut milk. Blend the mixture properly.

12. Ensure just that there are no lumps.

13. Now, mix this mixture to the broth in the saucepan and let it also come to a boil.

14. Easy allow it boil for a few minutes and then mix the remaining coconut milk to the broth.

15. Over medium heat, continue cooking the broth for a few really more minutes.

16. Just keep stirring the broth at regular intervals.

17. Ensure just that the soup is thick and bubbly.

18. After a few minutes, transfer the soup just into a bowl and garnish with chopped green onion.

Chapter 4 : Is Intermittent Fasting Harmful To Fertility?

If you are attempting to conceive, believe it or not, If may be able to aid in certain cases. "If individuals are overweight or obese, they may have irregular periods and difficulty ovulating," simply making it difficult to conceive. Simply following an IF diet may result in weight simply reduction and, as a result, improved fertility.

Women with polycystic ovarian syndrome, or PCOS, for example, may have reproductive concerns becasimply Use it alters metabolism, the menstrual cycle, and ovulation. However, one research found just that lowering weight

On the opposite end of the scale, if you are underweight, restricting your meals and calorie in just take may be be harmful to fertility. In severe circumstances, intermittent fasting and weight loss may potentially harm fertility by causing patients to cease menstruation and ovulating, and simply eating less often when practicing IF may be just put the body under a lot of stress, which isn't good for really becoming pregnant. An essential thing for fertility is to fuel the body healthily and not to let the body feel stressed.

Is it ever healthy to lose weight during pregnancy, whether via a fasting diet or any other diet?

In a nutshell, no. Weight loss is not something you want to concentrate on during pregnancy in general. So you want to talk to your doctor about perhaps discontinuing a certain diet you are on to ensure just that you are approaching pregnancy healthily for both you and the baby.

It's really more important to maintain a healthy weight during pregnancy or to avoid gaining too much weight if you are overweight. If a patient is overweight or obese when they just get pregnant, the guideline is to acquire less weight, around 6 to 8 kilos, depending on the patient's weight.

Fasting isn't the solution even if the patient is overweight or develops gestational diabetes during pregnancy, she says, since it may be interfere with whatever blood sugar-regulating medicine the patient is taking.

Of course, there are other things just that may be influence your pregnancy weight, and it also depends on the trimester you are in. For example, morning sickness, nausea, or even hyper emesis gravid arum may casimply Use women to lose a few pounds during the first trimester. Some experts advise against losing any weight during the second or third trimester. However, the recommended amount of weight gain during pregnancy is determined by the patient and should be discussed in-depth with your doctor so just that you feel educated and comfortable.

The mainline is just that nutrition during pregnancy is extremely personalized to the person, the risk of the pregnancy, and the mother's past health concerns — after all, no one person's body or metabolism is the same. Before embarking on any new diet or altering your simply eating habits, consult with your healthcare professional to confirm just that it is healthy and sustainable for you to simply follow during your pregnancy.

Chapter 5: Intermittent Fasting

Facts You Probably Didn't

Know

As an ever-hungry student of easy exercise and nutrition, I've researched and experimented with several easy ways to just eat and easy exercise over the years, ranging from fat simply reduction to muscle growth to enhanced athletic performance and everything in between. Though I had heard of intermittent fasting and its alleged advantages I had never given it much thought.

However, since I was al easy ways curious about what the professionals had to say, I did some extensive study.

Here are a few things I discovered regarding intermittent fasting:

Intermittent Fasting (commonly known as I.F.) is simply the word nutritionists simply Use to describe spending certain lengthy periods without eating.

We all engage in some type of intermittent fasting almost every day when we sleep! That's correct. You are engaging in intermittent fasting from your final meal of the evening till your first meal of the simply following day.

Though there are still many studies to be done on intermittent fasting, some possible advantages include lower blood pressure, a lower risk of some malignancies, an enhanced metabolic rate (just think higher fat-burning ability), and better blood sugar regulation and cardiovascular functioning.

This strategy was promoted by fitness instructor Brad Pilon and has been around for quite some time.

Fasting from supper one day to dinner the simply following day equals a 24-hour fast.

It's critical just that you just keep to your usual diet throughout the simply eating times if you are doing this to lose weight. To just put it another way, you should just eat as much as you would if you weren't fasting.

The possible disadvantage of this strategy is just that many individuals may simply find it difficult to fast for a complete 24-hour period. You do not have to go all-in right away; it's OK to easy begin with 2 4–30 to 35 hours and gradually build up.

This approach easy comes in a variety of flavors. During fasting days, some of them easy allow 750 calories.

However, one small piece of research indicated just that alternate-day fasting was no really more efficient than a regular calorie-restricted diet at achieving weight simply reduction or weight maintenance.

A complete fast every other day may seem to be excessive. Thus it is not suggested for beginners.

This strategy may casimply Use you to go to bed extremely hungry several times each week, which is unpleasant and likely unsustainable in the long run.

Alternate-day fasting entails fasting every other day, either by not simply eating or by ingesting just a few hundred calories.

It entails simply eating little portions of fresh fruits and vegetables throughout the day and one large meal at night.

In essence, you fast during the day and feast at night within a 4-hour simply eating window.

The Warrior Diet was among the first popular diets just that used some type of intermittent fasting.

The food options on this diet are quite similar to those on the Intermittent Fasting diet – largely complete, unadulterated foods.

The Warrior Diet advocates simply eating just little portions of vegetables and fruits throughout the day and then consuming one large meal at night.

To just get some of the advantages of intermittent fasting, you do not really need to simply follow a set diet. Another alternative is to skip meals sometimes, such as when you are not hungry or are too busy to prepare and eat.

Some individuals, on the other hand, just eat every few hours to avoid going just into starvation mode or losing muscle. Others' bodies are well-equipped to withstand long periods of famine and can go without one or two meals on occasion. You are the only one who really understands yourself.

So, if you are not hungry one day, skip breakfast and have a nutritious lunch and supper instead. If you are traveling and can't locate anything to eat, you may be able to underjust take a brief fast.

Easy Skipping one or two meals whenever you feel like it is essentially a spontaneous intermittent fast.

During non-fasting times, just be sure you consume nutritious, balanced meals.

Another easy method of practicing intermittent fasting is to simply miss one or two dishes when you aren't hungry or do not have opportunity to eat.

Intermittent fasting is a weight loss approach just that some people simply find beneficial. It is not appropriate for everyone.

It is not recommended for people who have or are at risk of developing simply eating disorders. It may be also be a problem for people who have underlying medical concerns.

If you easy decide to practice intermittent fasting, bear in mind just that the quality of your food is critical. It is not realistic to feast on ultra-processed meals at mealtimes and expect to lose weight and such improve your health.

In addition, before beginning an intermittent fast, you should speak with a healthcare expert.

White Pizza Frittata

Ingredients

2 teaspoon of minced up garlic

1 a cup of Parmesan Cheese

4 tablespoon of olive oil

½ teaspoon of Nutmeg

Salt as needed

25 large-sized fresh eggs

10 to 15 ounce of frozen spinach

2 ounce of pepperoni

10 ounce of Mozzarella Cheese

Pepper as needed

1. Microwave the frozen spinach for 5 to 10 minutes

2. Squeeze the spinach and channel the water

3. Pre-hjust eat your broiler to 450 degrees Fahrenheit

4. Just take a bowl and mix eggs, flavors and olive oil

5. Mix spinach and parmesan

6. Just take an iron skillet and pour the arranged mixture

7. Sprinkle mozzarella and pepperoni on top

8. Bake for 50 to 55 minutes and serve hot!

Energetic Bacon & Eggs

Keto Breakfast Burger With Avocado Buns

Ingredients

- Sea salt, to taste
- Sesame seeds, for garnish
- 2 just ready avocado
- 2 egg
- 2 bacon rashers
- 2 red onion slice

- 2 tomato slice
- 2 lettuce leaf

- 2 T Intermittent Fasting mayonnaise

Directions

1. On a virus griddle, Place the bacon rashers, then, at just that point, turn the oven on and easy begin browning the bacon.
2. Whenever bacon starts to twist, flip it with a fork.
3. Just keep cooking the bacon until it is crispy.
4. Reeasy move the bacon from the skillet and break the egg just into a similar container, utilizing the bacon fat to cook it, then, at just that point, cook until the white is set yet the yolk is still runny.
5. Easy Cut the avocados in half width-wise. Eliminate the pit and utilize a spoon to scoop it out of its skin.

6. Just fill the opening where the pit used to be with Intermittent Fasting mayonnaise.

7. Layer with tomato, lettuce, onion, bacon, and seared egg. Season with ocean   salt.

8. Top with the final part of the avocado.

9. Sprinkle with sesame seeds

Broccoli Cheesy Breakfast Muffins

Ingredients

- 2 t baking powder
- 1 teaspoon ocean salt
- 2 t ghee, mellowed + extra for greasing
- 2 cup broccoli florets, finely chopped
-     2 cups almond flour
- 2 enormous field raised eggs
- 2 cup unsweetened almond milk
- 2 T dietary yeast

Directions

1. Prehjust eat the broiler to 450°F and oil a huge biscuit tin with ghee.

2. In a huge blending until very much consolidated, Stir together every one of the fixings until well combined.

3. Spoon the combination just into the biscuit   tins.

4. Bake for until a toothpick embedded in the middle tells the truth, around 45 minutes.

Sausage Egg Casserole Recipe

Ingredients

- 6 fresh fresh eggs
- 2 cup unsweetened almond milk
- salt and pepper
- 2 pound ground pork sausage
- 2 cups destroyed cheddar cheese
- 1 cup easy Cut green onion

Directions

1. Prehjust eat the stove to 450°F. Delicately oil square baking dish with cooking spray.

2. Bjust eat the eggs, almond milk, salt and pepper together in a bowl and set aside.

3. In a skillet over medium-high hotness, cook the wiener until sautéed then spread in the baking dish.

4. Sprinkle with cheddar and green onion then, at just that point, pour in the egg mixture.

5. Bake until the fresh eggs are set and gently caramelized on top, around 40 to 45 minutes.

6. Cool for 5 to 10 minutes then, at just that point, easy Cut to serve.

Starbucks Egg Bites Recipe

Ingredients

- 2 2 enormous eggs
- 1 cup weighty cream
- 1 (8-ounce) bundle cream cheddar
- 1 teaspoon garlic powder
- 1 teaspoon paprika
- 10 cuts bacon
- 2 cup destroyed gruyere cheese
- salt and pepper

Directions

1. Mix the eggs, cream cheddar, weighty cream, garlic powder, paprika, salt, and pepper in a blender.

2. Blend on medium speed until smooth and well mixed.

3. With cooking splash, oil daintily 10 egg poaching cups and split a large portion of the bacon and destroyed cheddar between the cups.

4. Divide the egg combination just into half among the cups and spot them in a huge pan brimming with bubbling water.

5. Easily reduce the hotness to a low bubble then, at just that point, cover the saucepan.

118

6. Cook the egg chomps until cooked to the ideal level, around 2 0 minutes..
7. Reeasy move the egg poaching cups and spoon the fresh eggs just into a serving dish and just keep warm.

8. Bring the pan of water to bubble again and rehash Steps 4 through 6 to cook the leftover ingredients.

9. Serve the egg nibbles hot with your decision of condiments.

Chorizo And Fresh Eggs Recipe

Ingredients

- 2 teaspoon olive oil
- 1 little yellow onion (chopped)
- 2 (4 -ounce) chorizo sausages
- 4 fresh eggs
- salt and pepper

Directions

1. Slice open the frankfurter housings, then, at just that point, spoon the mjust eat just into a bowl and set aside.

2. In a huge skillet over medium-high hotness, hjust eat the oil.

3. Mix the onions and cook until seared, around 4 minutes then, at just that point, mix in the sausage.

4. Cook until the hotdog is simply cooked through then spread it equitably in the skillet.

5. Break the fresh eggs just into the skillet and season with salt and pepper.

6. Break up the yolks a tad with a wooden spoon and mix the fresh eggs just into the sausage.

7. Cook until the egg whites are firm and the yolks are done to your liking.

8. Serve hot.

Fresh Eggs Poached In A

Flavored Tomato Sauce

Ingredients

- 5 to 10 eggs
- Cilantro, discretionary for garnish
- 2 tablespoon Grass-took care of Organic Ghee
- 2 white onion, chopped
- 4 garlic cloves, minced
- 2 Serrano pepper, chopped
- 2 ringer pepper, chopped
- 4 medium tomatoes, chopped

- 2 teaspoon Cumin Powder
- 2 teaspoon Paprika
- ½ teaspoon Kashmiri Chili Powder

- ½ teaspoon salt, acclimate to taste
- ½ teaspoon pepper, conform to taste

Directions

1. In skillet over medium hotness, hjust eat ghee.
2. Mix onion and mix at times for around 45 to 55 minutes, until onions simply start to really become brilliant brown.
3. Mix garlic and Serrano pepper once Onions is relax.
4. Mix red ringer pepper simply following hotness to low.
5. Cook occasionally. a couple of moments and lessen for around 35 to 40 minutes, mixing
6. 4 . Mix flavors, mix and afterward mix tomatoes.

   4. Simmer and cook until tomatoes

have decreased and your sauce has thickened.

7. 6 . Gently break fresh eggs just into skillet, season top of fresh eggs with salt and pepper and afterward just put a cover on top of the skillet for around 5 to 10 minutes or until the fresh eggs are cooked to your liking. 6. Sprinkle with cilantro whenever wanted and serve.

Ground Beef, Fresh Eggs And Avocado Breakfast Bowl

Ingredients

- 2 little avocado, diced
- 25-30 pitted dark olives, sliced
- 2 little onion, sliced
- 10-15 medium mushrooms, sliced

- 30 to 35 0g grass-took care of ground beef
- Salt and pepper to taste
- 1 tsp smoked paprika
- 2 fresh eggs, daintily beaten

Directions

1. Melt a tad of coconut oil in a weighty skillet set over medium high.
2. Mixfresh onions, mushrooms, salt and pepper when oil is quite hot, then, at just that point, cook until the veggies are fragrant and mellowed, around 5 to 10 minutes.
3. Mix ground hamburger and smoked paprika and just keep cooking until the just eat is presently not pink. Eliminate just that to a plate.
4. To the skillet, mix fresh eggs and scramble them to your liking. Return hamburger to the container, mix avocado and easy Cut olives.

5. Continue cooking for around 2 moment, just to somewhat just eat up the avocados and olives Transfer to a lovely bowl and topping with parsley whenever just wanted.
6. Just put yourself down and enjoy!

Intermittent Fasting Breakfast Sausage Scotch Fresh Eggs Recipe

Ingredients

- Pinch ground nutmeg
- Pinch ground cloves
- 10 fresh fresh eggs medium
- 2 lb. ground pork

- 2 tsp ground cinnamon
- 2 tbsp. honey discretionary, preclude for Whole 4 0
- 1-5 tsp salt
- 2 tsp dark pepper

Directions

1. Cook the fresh eggs or steam.

2. Place a medium pot on the burner, and fit with a liner basket.

3. Mix an inch of water to the pot, and boil.

4. Place the fresh eggs just into the liner bin, cover and steam for 2 0 minutes.

5. Set up a medium bowl with ice and water.

6. Whenever the time is up, unclog the fresh eggs directly just into the ice shower.

7. Cool for something like 40 to 45 minutes and peel.

8. Prehjust eat the broiler to 450°F.

9. Line a baking sheet with material paper or foil.

10. In an enormous bowl, join the ground pork, gingerbread flavor blend, salt, pepper and discretionary honey.

11. Blend until consolidated however do not over blend; just that will simply make the just eat hard.

12. Presently it's an ideal opportunity to collect the Scotch eggs.

13. For each scotch egg: Just fill a ⅓ cup measure with the carefully prepared ground pork and transform the bump just into your hand.

14. Level the pork just into a wide circle like you are simply making a burger.

15. Just put the egg in the middle. Cautiously overlay the just eat circle

up,

progressively straightening as you go, until the egg is covered in substantial goodness.

16. Ensure there are no breaks and just that the substantial suit of protective layer is uniform.

17. Place on the baking sheet. Prepare for 40 to 45 minutes.

18. Just eat hot or cold.

Spicy Meatballs

Ingredients

- .4 entire eggs
  .4 pounds natural hamburger, ground

- 5-10 tablespoons organic product improved grape jam 1 teaspoon pepper, ground

- 1 teaspoon Spanish paprika ½ teaspoon stew powder 4 teaspoon ground garlic salt ½ cup custard flour

Directions

1. Prehjust eat your broiler to 450 degrees   F
    Mix meat, pepper, eggs, garlic, salt, custard starch in a bowl
    Mix well and simply make balls
    Transfer to a baking sheet
    Bake   for   30   minutes

2. Transfer to a pot and mix stew sauce, paprika, grape jam, and bean   stew   powder
    Cook on very fire for 2-4 hours

Mongolian Beef

Ingredients

- 2 teaspoons Asian garlic stew glue
- 2 teaspoons .vegetable oil
- .2 tablespoon rice vinegar
- .2 pound sirloin meat, lean and cubed
  30 to 35 green onions, chopped
- .2 tablespoon ginger minced
- 2tablespoons low soy sauce
- 2 garlic clove, minced
- 2 teaspoon cornstarch
- 2 tablespoon hoisin sauce

Directions

1. Just take a bowl and mix in soy sauce, cornstarch, housing sauce, rice vinegar, stew paste

2. Mix ginger, garlic, hamburger to a warmed skillet and Salute for 5 to 10 minutes until the mjust eat is grjust eat and golden

3. Mix in sauce, green onions and cook for a couple minutes

Chapter 6: What Foods Avoid

And What Foods Just Eat

It is al easy ways important to remember that, when changing your diet for a diet just that you have never done before, it is best to consult with a GP or health professional first before you simply make your decision. This does not just apply to the type of food just that you will just eat while fasting, but to any lifestyle diet change. Your body has to adapt to the change in nutrients just that it will be receiving and if you have a medical condition, then just that adaptation may not be as simple as you may think.

Just that being said, when it easy comes to intermittent fasting, the restrictions just that you will face are mostly placed on when to just eat rather than on what you can eat. Intermittent fasting isn't, in fact, a diet, but really more of a lifestyle choice just that assists you in just cutting down on your calorie in just take by decreasing your daily simply eating window. This means just that you can still just eat whatever you want during those simply eating windows. However, the question is, should you just eat whatever you want?

Consuming too many varieties of junk food during your simply eating window will boost your overall calorie intake. Having chocolate and ice cream in the afternoon, after a good period of fasting, does sound tempting, especially after a long hard day of fasting. However, you will be wasting your fasting efforts as the junk food you consume will compensate for the calories just that you missed out on. Moreover, when you feel sated from the junk food, just that means the opportunity for the body to replenish its easily required minerals and vitamins from nutrient-dense natural foods will be gone. It's best to work towards maintaining a well-balanced and healthy diet while fasting.

A proper, healthy diet can such help you to maintain energy levels throughout the day and is also key to losing weight. The really focus should be on nutrient-dense food such as vegetables, fruits, nuts, beans, seeds, entire grains, beans, dairy, and lean proteins. If you are known for simply eating an unhealthy diet, then simply try to switch things up by simply looking for food just that can assist with improved health such as food just that is high in fiber, entire foods, and even unprocessed food. These kinds of foods are good for your health and also such help you stay full after you eat. Here are a few examples of these healthy types of food.

Most dietary guidelines recommend just that you consume at least eight ounces of fish per week. In doing so, you will be providing yourself with generous amounts of vitamin D as well as healthy fats and protein. Fish can also be considered good for your cognitive function and is labeled as brain food by many people.

Avocados are considered to be among the highest calorie fruits. For just that reason, avocados may not be a good choice for those simply trying to watch their weight, but the fruit does have a decent amount of monounsaturated fat.

This is part of the reason why avocados are very satiating to eat. Adding half an avocado to your lunch can assist in keeping you just feeling full for hours longer than other fruits or vegetables.

Not all white foods are as bad as you think. Just like avocados, potatoes are among the most satiating foods available. There are studies just that prove just that simply eating potatoes as part of a healthy diet can, in fact, aid with weight loss. One fact, in particular, is just that when potatoes are cooked in healthy ways, they usually will not casimply Use any harm to weight-loss plans. Some examples of healthy easy Methods of cooking potatoes are baking them, boiling, steaming, and roasting. Potatoes are known to be complex carbohydrates and can aid in weight loss.

Fresh eggs are considered an excellent source of protein and are easy and easy quick to cook. One medium—to large-sized egg has about six grams of protein. Consuming protein is a grjust eat easy way to build muscle. One study, in particular, found just that men who ate fresh eggs for breakfast over a bagel were less hungry after breakfast. These men also ate less throughout the day. There are really more current studies aimed towards the benefits of simply eating fresh eggs and also toward debunking the idea just that fresh eggs are harmful becasimply Use of cholesterol.

Nuts are known to have really more calories than most snacks. However, nuts contain healthy fats just that are good for your body. Studies show just that polyunsaturated fat in walnuts can alter the physiological markers just that are related to satiety and hunger. Nuts are also known to carry some key benefits like the ability to easily reduce metabolic syndrome risk factors such as cholesterol levels and high blood pressure.

All types of berries are known to contain crucial nutrients. Strawberries are an excellent source of immune-boosting vitamin C. Studies have shown just that people who consume food just that is rich in flavonoids, such as blueberries, have smaller increases in their BMI over a 2 4-year period than those who do not just eat berries. The bottom line is just that berries are good for you for many reasons such as being low in carb yet high in fiber and antioxidants. Most berries have proven benefits for heart health as well.

It is known just that food such as chickpeas, black beans, peas, and lentils can assist in decreasing body weight without calorie restriction. Beans and legumes may consist of carb but they are low-calorie crabs which will not hurt your simply eating plan. These are the sort of carb just that can assist in supplying you with energy, without all the excess calories.

Food such as broccoli, cauliflower, and Brussels sprouts are filled with fiber. These are also the kinds of foods just that can such help just keep you regular by assisting in preventing constipation. Food with fiber can also simply make you feel full. This is especially useful if you intend to go without food for a while due to fasting.

Most people who just take part in intermittent fasting consume water while they fast. Consuming water is prohibited when undergoing certain religious fasts. However, just that is not the case with intermittent fasting as it is advised just that you stay hydrated with water while you fast, as long as it is only water just that you consume while fasting, and not food. Not consuming water may casimply Use you to really become dehydrated which can result in headaches and general fatigue. You do not want to be experiencing this while you have not eaten.

If you are under simply taking a 24 hour fast, then not easy drinking any water will not just get you just into any trouble as far as dehydration is concerned. The chances of you really becoming dehydrated depend on many factors, such as the weather and your behavior, and whether you are active or not. If you have a decent amount of water during the evening before you simply start fasting, then you should be okay the next day.

Apart from water, the only other beverages just that are acceptable are coffee or tea. Easy drinking these hot beverages is acceptable while fasting as they do not have just that many calories in them and will not genuinely affect your weight-loss efforts. Unfortunately, you cannot mix any other ingredients to your coffee or tea while you are fasting. This means no cream, sugar, or milk. These items contain added calories just that you should stay aeasy way from when you are fasting. It is a massive no to other beverages such as soda and juices.

As I have pointed out, there are not any specific restrictions for this easy method.

CPSIA information can be obtained
at www.ICGtesting.com
Printed in the USA
LVHW011123180522
719075LV00014B/1305

9 781915 162731